Teachers of Healing and Wholeness

Patanjali

Also in this series

1 · ANDREW BOORDE: HEALING THROUGH MIRTH

2 · HIPPOCRATES: THE NATURAL REGIMEN

3 · HUANG DI: THE BALANCE OF YIN AND YANG

Other titles in preparation

Teachers of Healing and Wholeness

Patanjali
The Threads of Yoga

ARTHUR JAMES
BERKHAMSTED

First published in Great Britain by
ARTHUR JAMES LTD
70 Cross Oak Road
Berkhamsted
Hertfordshire HP4 3HZ

Introduction and selection:
© Robert Van de Weyer 1997

All rights reserved. No part of this book may be reproduced, stored in a retrieval system, or transmitted by any means, electronic, mechanical, photocopying, recording, or otherwise, without the prior written permission of the publishers.

This book is sold subject to the condition that it shall not, by way of trade or otherwise, be lent, re-sold, hired out or otherwise circulated without the publisher's prior consent in any form of binding or cover other than that in which it is published and without a similar condition including this condition being imposed on the subsequent purchaser.

A catalogue record for this book is available from the British Library.

ISBN 0 85305 413 4

Typeset in Monotype Columbus by
Strathmore Publishing Services, London N7

Printed in Great Britain at
Ipswich Book Company, Ipswich, Suffolk

Contents

	Series Introduction	vii
	Introduction	ix
1	The Purpose of Yoga	1
2	The Way of Yoga	12
3	The Method of Yoga	24
4	The Summary of Yoga	31
	Bibliography	36

Series Introduction

At a time when the limitations of modern medicine are becoming clear, growing numbers of people are looking back to older approaches to healing and wholeness. The series aims to make available to the general reader original writings of the great teachers, from every part of the world and from every period of history.

The particular insights of the different teachers vary, and each has special wisdom for us to hear. Yet various themes recur. They all stress the unity of the spiritual and physical aspects of human nature, and therefore the need to care for the whole person. They emphasise the importance of the way we conduct our daily lives, both to prevent and to cure illness. And they seek to harness the latent powers of self-healing.

None of the healers in this series claimed to be infallible; all saw themselves as explorers. Thus none asked for uncritical trust; they regarded themselves as partners with those who listened to their words. In reading their works today we should see ourselves as partners, reflecting on what they say, and taking such advice as we think is right.

Introduction

The most famous contribution of the Hindu religion to the world is the practice of Yoga. And the greatest teacher of Yoga was Patanjali, who lived about two thousand years ago. His series of aphorisms describe the state of perfect mental harmony, and show how through meditation this state can be attained. The aphorisms are also intended as foci for meditation, and thus are themselves aids in the practice of Yoga.

The word Yoga literally means union; and it is used in Hinduism to describe every aspect of religion and morality which promotes unity within the individual, and between the individual and other living creatures. Patanjali used the term more specifically as the name for a particular mental and physical discipline. The central element of this discipline is meditation, in which the mind fixes itself on a particular object or sound; and through regular meditation the mind gradually becomes serene and tranquil, free from all disturbance. This in turn raises the soul to what Patanjali calls 'superior consciousness' in which all distinctions of time and space, pleasure and pain, disappear.

Some traditions of Yoga complement meditation with highly complex physical exercises; indeed these physical exercises can be helpful in themselves, quite apart from meditation. Patanjali, however, makes only two stipulations about the body. Firstly the practitioner of Yoga should have a firm and healthy posture, in which no pain or discomfort is experienced. Secondly breathing should be deep and calm.

The aphorisms of Patanjali are called 'sutras,' which means threads. And they are written not as a series of instructions, but rather as a number of threads which are woven together to form a pattern. Thus they do not follow logically one to the next; and, more importantly, they are not intended to be understood by the logical part of the mind. Initially they should be read as a whole, to give a general indication of the nature and purpose of Yoga. Then those who begin to practise meditation should take particular aphorisms, and fix their minds on them; in this way their inner meaning becomes clear. Eventually the aphorisms are superceded by experience, and become unnecessary.

Patanjali does not demand an act of faith; he simply invites people to try Yoga, and gauge its effects for themselves. Over the centuries it has proved its worth. It is not a cure for particular mental or physical illnesses. But it is a means of overcoming the mental anxieties and disturbances that beset all people, and

INTRODUCTION

attaining a greater degree of inner peace. Few people reach a full state of superior consciousness; but every step in this direction brings benefits.

Nothing is known about Patanjali as a person. The earliest edition of his aphorisms in their present form appeared in the fourth century CE; but this was probably based on an earlier work, which may have been written two or three centuries previously. And Patanjali was himself not the originator of the practice he describes, but merely its codifier. Yet this obscurity is appropriate: Yoga seeks to dissolve the barriers between one individual and another, and between one period of history and another.

I

The Purpose of Yoga

The Purpose of Yoga

1. Let us explain Yoga:

2. Yoga is concerned with freedom from mental disturbances.

3. In this way the spirit becomes perfectly serene.

Disturbances to the Spirit

4 Without Yoga the spirit is in constant turmoil.

5 There are five kinds of disturbance, some painful, and some not painful.

6 These are: observation, doubt, idealism, pessimism, and memory.

7 By observation we mean perceiving external objects, drawing inferences about them; and learning about them from others.

8 By doubt we mean concern about the possibility that something may be different from what it appears.

9 By idealism we mean the external goals or ambitions which we set ourselves.

10 By pessimism we mean an outlook which regards evil as genuine.

11 By memory we mean attributing to external objects continuing and indefinite reality.

THE PURPOSE OF YOGA

Conditions for Freedom

12 To become free from mental disturbances requires effort and patience.

13 By effort we mean persistent attempts to attain serenity.

14 Persistence implies constant and uninterrupted devotion.

15 By patience we mean willingness gradually to relinquish all attachment to external objects, both seen and heard.

16 This willingness implies an acceptance of one's fate, whatever it may be.

Forms of Consciousness

17 Normal consciousness is concerned with reasoning, distinguishing one object from another, enjoyment and self-awareness.

18 There is also superior consciousness, in which all mental activity ceases; this is attained through various stages.

Superior Consciousness

19 Some have a natural tendency towards superior consciousness, which they have inherited from their forbears.

20 Others must attain superior consciousness through strong conviction, intense effort, deep study, firm concentration, and profound spiritual discernment.

21 Those who are most earnest are most likely to succeed in attaining superior consciousness.

22 The rate of progress depends on whether a person is mildly earnest, moderately earnest, or extremely earnest.

23 Those who wish to attain superior consciousness should seek and emulate an ideal soul.

24 An ideal soul is one who is unmoved by physical temptations, by promises of reward, and by bodily cravings.

25 In the ideal soul knowledge is at its highest level.

26 The ideal soul is symbolised by the sound AUM.

27 Repetition of AUM, and understanding of its significance, helps towards the attainment of superior consciousness.

Obstacles in Yoga

28 In moving from normal consciousness towards superior consciousness, there are various obstacles to be overcome.

29 These obstacles include laziness, uncertainty of purpose, lack of enthusiasm, lethargy, sensuality, belief in the reality of the material world, and failure to maintain a strict routine in practising Yoga.

30 Alongside these obstacles we add depression, anxiety, bodily restlessness, and troublesome breathing.

The Steady Mind

31 Overcoming these obstacles requires single-minded effort.

32 Single-minded effort is helped by having supportive friends, by looking upon all people with good will, and by being indifferent to success and failure.

33 Single-mindedness is also attained by steady and relaxed breathing.

34 Meditation on a plant is a means of steadying the mind.

35 Meditation on a light may also steady the mind.

36 Meditation on an inanimate object can be helpful too.

37 Some find it easiest to hold their attention steady when they are in a dreamy or sleepy state.

38 It is a matter of personal choice as to how the mind is kept steady.

39 The mind which is meditating becomes indifferent to the size of objects, from the tiniest to the largest.

The Perceiver and the Perceived

⁴⁰ Once a steady mind has been attained, it is time to consider the relationship between the perceiver and the object perceived.

⁴¹ The relationship between the perceiver and the object perceived is also connected with the words used by perceivers to describe objects.

⁴² The relationship is connected with the issue of observation: what inferences the mind has drawn about the object perceived.

⁴³ The relationship is connected with the issue of doubt: whether the object perceived is the same as, or different from, how it appears.

⁴⁴ Observation and doubt disturb the steady mind; so the relationship between the perceiver and the object perceived must exclude them.

THE PURPOSE OF YOGA

Freedom from Desire

⁴⁵ So far we have considered the results which we desire from Yoga.

⁴⁶ But only when consciousness is freed from all desire does the true nature of things become clear.

⁴⁷ Free from desire, the mind sees through the veil of appearance, and becomes aware of reality.

⁴⁸ Ordinary knowledge, obtained through observation and inference, sees only particular truths about things.

⁴⁹ The mind that is free from desire must not even desire the awareness which such freedom brings.

⁵⁰ Freedom from desire yields true enjoyment in the mind.

2
The Way of Yoga

The Five Hindrances

1. In order to practise Yoga you should learn to control yourself, and to understand yourself.

2. The aim of Yoga is the attainment of inner harmony, by breaking down the barriers which hinder it.

3. There are five hindrances to harmony: ignorance, egoism, attachment, aversion, and tenacity.

4. Ignorance is the soil in which the other hindrances grow.

5. Ignorance consists in mistaking the transient for the eternal, the impure for the pure, evil for good, the apparent self for the real self.

6. Egoism consists in identifying the soul, which is the source of awareness, with the instruments of awareness, which are the senses and the mind.

7 Attachment consists in being tied to the causes of pleasure.

8 Aversion consists in being fearful of the causes of pain.

9 Tenacity consists in clinging to bodily life.

10 These five hindrances can gradually be overcome by persistent effort.

11 This effort can only be properly directed if you recognise the hindrances within yourself.

12 Every thought and action either strengthens or weakens the hindrances.

13 So long as the hindrances remain, they determine your roles in life, the length of your life, and the joys and sorrows you experience through life.

14 Joy is the fruit of thoughts and actions that weaken hindrances; and sorrow is the fruit of thoughts and actions that strengthen hindrances.

15 Yet even at moments of joy there will always be inner turmoil, until full unity has been attained.

16 If you practise Yoga, the duration and depth of that turmoil is progressively reduced.

The Association of Soul and Body

17 The underlying reason why you do not experience inner harmony is the association of the soul, the source of awareness, with the objects of awareness.

18 Awareness of external objects starts with the senses, and leads from the senses to the mind; it then causes either action or inertia.

19 The mind becomes aware of objects as well-defined, ill-defined, or merely implied by signs.

20 Awareness leads from the mind to the soul.

21 The mind and the senses only function because the soul is present.

22 When the soul is liberated, and attains harmony, it transcends awareness; yet for other souls, who are not yet liberated, the objects of awareness continue to exist.

23 Association of the soul and body makes it appear to the soul that it possesses a body, and to the body that it possesses a soul.

24 But the appearance is illusory.

25 When the illusion of the soul possessing a body, and the body possessing a soul, disappears, the association of the soul and body ceases. The soul is liberated from the body, and is free.

26 The way to shatter this illusion is through continuous effort at discerning reality.

27 By shattering the illusion the soul moves upwards from normal to superior consciousness.

The Eight Stages

28 In order to discern reality, you must proceed gradually through the eight stages of Yogic practice.

29 The eight stages are: abstinence, devotion, right posture, right breathing, retracting the senses, fixing the attention, fusion of awareness and objects, inner harmony.

The Five Abstinences

30 The person wishing to practise Yoga must abstain from: injuring other people or any other living creatures, speaking dishonestly and giving false impressions, taking things that belong to other people or any other living creatures, becoming attached to particular pleasures and their causes, becoming attached to particular external objects.

31 These abstinences are universal, and must be practised in all places, times and circumstances, and in every aspect of your life.

The Five Devotions

32 The person wishing to practise Yoga must be devoted to: cleanliness, both inward and outward; serenity, self-control, self-knowledge, and to the ideal of superior consciousness.

33 Abstinence and devotion go together, since abstinence from that which is evil implies devotion to that which is good.

34 Failure to observe the five abstinences may be deliberate or unintentional, it may be prompted by anger or by thoughtlessness, it may be slight or it may be great. But every failure causes inner turmoil.

35 Enmity between yourself and other people, and between yourself and other kinds of living creature, only ceases when the desire to cause injury ceases.

36 You can only learn to be honest with yourself, if you no longer wish to deceive other people.

37 When you no longer desire to take things that belong to others, then you realise that all things belong to everyone and no one.

38 When you are attached to no external objects, your spiritual energy multiplies.

39 Once the drive to possess things has been uprooted, then you can perceive their inner reality.

40 When you are clean, both inwardly and outwardly, you are no longer concerned about your external appearance, nor about other people's opinion of you.

41 Inner and outer cleanliness leads to serenity, cheerfulness, concentration of the mind, control of the senses, and spiritual insight.

42 From serenity flows great enjoyment of life.

43 From self-control flows awareness of the body and its organs.

44 Self-knowledge leads you to realise that you can only achieve fulfilment through attaining superior consciousness.

45 If you can imagine yourself in an ideal state of superior consciousness, then you will want, above all, to attain that state.

Right posture

46 The right posture is firm and comfortable.

47 Right posture comes from reducing the tendency towards restlessness.

48 Restlessness of the body arises from tensions in the mind. These tensions must be eased.

Right Breathing

49 Right breathing depends on controlling the motions of inhaling and exhaling.

50 You are breathing badly if your inhalations are too shallow, and your exhalations too rapid.

51 When you are breathing badly, your mind is constantly being disturbed.

52 When you breathe easily and freely, your mind becomes more peaceful.

53 When you breathe easily and freely, you are better able to concentrate the mind.

Retracting the Senses

⁵⁴ Retracting the senses means paying no more attention to objects of pleasure than to any other objects.

⁵⁵ This requires complete control of the senses.

3
The Method of Yoga

Fixing the Attention

1. Meditation begins by fixing the attention to some particular object.

2. Your attention and the external object become fused.

3. The mind thus becomes unconscious of itself.

4. As a result all mental disturbance ceases, and the mind experiences harmony within itself.

5. Gradually the light of true knowledge enters the mind.

6. No effort should be made to make this light brighter; it should be allowed to grow brighter in stages.

7. Although the mind has fused with an external object, the source of this fusion is within.

THE METHOD OF YOGA

8. And this source itself has no origin; it is its own source.

9. The desire to suppress mental disturbance must also be suppressed, because all desire is a cause of mental disturbance.

10. The mind is only truly free from disturbance when the desire to suppress disturbance has itself been suppressed.

11. As inner harmony is attained, the mind no longer regards itself as a distinct entity.

12. As the mind ceases to see itself as a distinct entity, it also ceases to make a distinction between harmony and disturbance.

13. The mind knows itself and the body perfectly; yet it does not know itself or the body at all.

14. All things have periods of disturbance, and periods of harmony.

15. Progress in Yoga reduces the periods of disturbance, and lengthens the periods of harmony.

Mental Harmony

16 In a state of inner harmony, the mind ceases to distinguish between past and future; they are perceived as one.

17 Words make distinctions between entities. In a state of inner harmony, in which all things are perceived as one, words lose their meaning.

18 The attainment of mental harmony is the means by which a person rises to superior consciousness.

19 Through mental harmony, in which distinctions cease, the mind is able to apprehend the thoughts of other minds.

20 The harmonious mind can perceive clearly the attachments which disturb other minds.

21 The five senses are heightened and clarified through mental harmony, because the mind is not disturbed by what the senses perceive.

THE METHOD OF YOGA

22 Through mental harmony the distinction between actions which are intended, and those which are unintended, disappears. This is because a harmonious mind can always anticipate the effects of the actions which it prompts.

23 The person whose mind is in harmony is consistently friendly towards others.

24 The person whose mind is in harmony has no wish to exercise power over others.

25 The harmonious mind is extremely observant, because no disturbance interferes with its observations.

26 By fixing its attention on one thing, the harmonious mind understands all things.

27 By contemplating the moon, the harmonious mind understands the stars.

28 By contemplating the sun, the harmonious mind understands the universe.

29 By contemplating the navel, the harmonious mind understands the entire body.

30 By contemplating the throat, the harmonious mind understands hunger and thirst, and can control them.

31 By contemplating the blinking of the eyes, the harmonious mind understands that motion and stillness are ultimately the same.

32 By contemplating its own inner light, the harmonious mind understands the nature of true knowledge.

33 The harmonious mind ceases to use logic as a means of understanding; intuition is sufficient, superseding logic.

34 The harmonious mind is not swayed by emotion, nor does it control the emotions; mind and heart are perfectly unified.

35 The mind makes itself harmonious not for its own sake, but for the sake of the soul.

36 The harmonious mind is never impressed by what it receives from the five senses.

THE METHOD OF YOGA

37 If the harmonious mind were impressed by what it received from the sense organs, it would lose its harmony.

38 The harmonious mind is free from slavery to the body.

39 This freedom means that bodily hunger and thirst cannot disturb it.

40 The harmonious mind is always at one with itself.

41 Sound and silence become one.

42 Body and space beyond the body become one.

43 Senses and the objects they perceive become one.

44 Largeness and smallness become one.

45 That which to the disturbed mind is gross is to the harmonious mind graceful.

46 That which the disturbed mind regards as ugly is to the harmonious mind beautiful.

47 The harmonious mind thinks without effort.

48 The harmonious mind knows itself.

49 Harmony of the mind leads to superior consciousness in the soul.

50 The harmonious mind allows the soul to rise upwards.

51 The soul derives no satisfaction from rising upwards because the distinction between satisfaction and dissatisfaction has ceased.

52 Time is no longer a line, in which one moment follows another.

53 Space no longer separates one thing from another.

54 The soul which has attained superior consciousness is both totally isolated, and also unified with all other souls.

55 The harmonious mind, and the soul in superior consciousness, are equally pure and equally perfect.

A Summary of Yoga

1. Success in Yoga is helped by innate ability, eating the right food, by thinking and acting in a loving manner towards other people, by having a regular routine, and by living quietly.

2. Within each human being every level of animate existence is simultaneously present.

3. A human being contains the nature of an insect, a reptile, a bird and an animal.

4. Once human beings come to know and love themselves, they come to know and love all living creatures.

5. Although the human mind can know and love many people and many other creatures, it remains one mind.

6. Practitioners of Yoga can never harm those whom they know.

7 In itself the practice of Yoga does not have good consequences, except for the practitioners themselves.

8 But the practitioners are quick to discern opportunities to do good to others.

9 By doing good to others, practitioners find that their mental harmony is enhanced.

10 Practitioners wish to do good, but do not derive pleasure from it.

11 Those who regularly do good to others get into the habit of good works, and thus can perform them without effort.

12 Since the past determines the future, past and future are not separate, but unified.

13 The future cannot escape the consequences of the past.

14 The substance of an object or a creature is that which does not change over time.

15 The substance of a human mind is that which cannot change.

16 A mind does not depend on the objects it perceives.

17 Objects do not depend on minds perceiving them.

18 An object may be known or unknown, depending on whether a mind perceives it.

19 A mind is always known, since it perceives itself.

20 The mind does not create its own awareness; the mind's awareness derives from the soul.

21 Through Yoga the mind simultaneously becomes aware of itself, and ceases to be aware of itself.

22 The mind ceases to become aware of itself because all distinctions between the mind and objects of awareness cease.

23 The mind which practises Yoga finds all objects and sounds interesting.

24 The mind which practises Yoga is disinterested in all objects and sounds.

25 Those who can discern the distinction between mind and soul no longer confuse the two.

26 The supreme object of attention for the mind is the soul.

27 When the mind meditates upon the soul, it becomes completely isolated from the physical world.

28 This isolation means that it cannot be disturbed by sense perceptions of the physical world.

29 The isolated mind cannot be disturbed by desire, because it cannot know desire.

30 The isolated mind cannot be disturbed by fear, because fear arises from events outside the mind.

31 The isolated mind knows everything, and yet knows nothing.

32 When the senses no longer affect the mind, they perceive the physical world with perfect clarity, and yet they do not perceive it at all.

33. The isolated mind functions perfectly, and ceases to function.

34. The soul is now pure. AUM

Bibliography

Bahm, A. J., *The Yoga Sutras of Patanjali*. Asian Humanities Press, Berkeley, 1961

Vivekananda, Swami, *The Yoga Aphorisms of Patanjali*. Ramakrishna Center, New York, 1953